A DEMENTIA CAREGIVER CALLED TO ACTION

The Journey

Dr. Macie P. Smith
Licensed Gerontology Social Worker
©2024 Dr. Macie P. Smith Publishing
Columbia, SC

The opinions and views uniquely expressed in this book are those of Dr. Macie P. Smith and are based on her years of research and experience, both professionally and personally, and should not be used in lieu of medical care or medical advice. The information in this book is not intended to be a substitute for professional medical advice, diagnosis or treatment. Always seek the advice of your physician or other qualified health provider with any questions you may have regarding a medical condition. Never disregard professional medical advice or delay in seeking it because of something you have read in this book. If you think you may have a medical emergency, call your doctor or 911 immediately.

Dr. Macie P. Smith does not recommend or endorse any specific tests, physicians, products, procedures, opinions or other information that may be mentioned in this book. Reliance on any information provided by Dr. Macie P. Smith, Dr. Smith's employees, others contributing to this book at the invitation of Dr. Smith or other patrons of this book is solely at your own risk. In no event shall Dr. Macie P. Smith, its content providers, its suppliers or any third parties mentioned in this book be liable for any claims or damages (including, without limitation, direct, incidental and consequential damages, personal injury/wrongful death or lost profits) resulting from the use of or inability to use the information in this book, whether based on warranty, contract, tort or any other legal theory, and whether or not Dr. Macie P. Smith is advised of the possibility of such damages.

Table of Contents

Impetus

If you are reading this book, you are likely aware that dementia is a growing health concern. Worldwide, more than 47 million people are living with some form of dementia. Alzheimer's disease accounts for approximately 60% of these cases. Currently, more than 6 million Americans are living with Alzheimer's disease. Approximately 38% are over the age of 85, 59% are over the age of 65 and 3.2 million are women. According to the Alzheimer's Association, women are at higher risk of developing Alzheimer's disease; they are also more likely to be caregivers. Statistics show that over 16 million caregivers are providing more than 18 billion hours of unpaid care for people living with dementia. Based on these numbers alone, it is clear family caregiving is one of the most crucial concerns facing our society today. Sadly, social policy is lagging in addressing this concern. Until a time when social policy catches up, this book will provide invaluable information to help you develop your own social support system and strategies along the dementia care journey.

Introduction

Because we know that many people living with dementia are being cared for by family members or loved ones in their community, there is a desperate need for community dementia education programs and comprehensive care. When we think of comprehensive care, we think of doctors collaborating with other doctors to support the patient's care in a dementia-specific holistic manner. But realistically speaking, all of the patients' physicians may not convene to discuss that patient's care. This fragmented approach to caring for people with dementia is not only unproductive, but it could have major implications for the person living with dementia and their family caregivers. Family caregivers have reported high levels of stress associated with family caregiving. This factor alone can lead to increased healthcare costs for family caregivers, leaving their loved ones with dementia at risk for placement in an assisted living or nursing facility.

Emerging research suggests that there is not a cure for Alzheimer's, the most common cause/type of dementia; however, there are medications that could manage the symptoms for a period of time. These include memory loss, confusion, mood changes, disorientation, lack of decision-making skills and compulsive behavior. As the disease progresses, so does the likelihood that these symptoms could worsen – with the bulk of the responsibility to manage the behaviors resting upon the family caregivers and other members of the extended family. Therefore, there is a growing need for dementia-competent education that is practical, applicable and relatable. From how dementia progresses to what resources are available, access to information and support services will go a long way to help ease or alleviate the high levels of stress the caregiver experiences.

As the number of people living with dementia continues to increase, so does the number of family caregivers. What the medical profession is now realizing is that people who develop irreversible dementia will eventually depend on someone to manage and coordinate their care as the condition progresses.

As a result of this budding crisis, physician practices are now faced with the responsibility of managing the care of people living with dementia as well as their caregiver(s); in essence, at least two patients now exist. As it stands, general practitioners are not familiar with the many home and community based services that are now available to aid in the person's ability to safely remain in their natural environment for as long as feasibly possible, e.g. in-home care aide, respite and environmental modification. Therefore, doctors' offices must make a conscious effort to seek out sources of information and education that encompass non-pharmacological strategies since the medical model is only a small piece of the puzzle. Physicians also must learn more about home and community-based options that are designed to assist the aging population age in place safely. Nursing homes are no longer the only option today; and in some cases, it is not an option at all when considering its price tag.

People living with a progressive form of dementia must have a team of professionals talking to each other on a regular basis about the person's medical care, social care, and community care in order to ensure quality of life. It is because of this unique need that professional Geriatric Care Management is now considered a mainstream service that is an integral component in providing competent, quality, individualized and respectful care for people living with dementia.

Geriatric Care Management is a growing field comprised of professionals who help senior families cope with the medical and social complexities of aging by developing care strategies that allow older people to remain independent for as long as possible and to assist in arranging for and assuring the quality of long-term care as appropriate to meet individual needs. Geriatric Care Managers are integral in providing expertise in areas that are time consuming or inappropriate for an attorney or a physician. For example, a Geriatric Care Manager can evaluate a senior's home environment and make suggestions based on the senior's physical, social, and medical needs. It is the responsibility of the Geriatric Care

Manager to be knowledgeable of the available resources in the community to assist the senior family with their daily needs.

Medical practices need social workers and community health workers now more than ever to help manage the amount of care and support that people living with dementia require. An ongoing dementia-specific care plan needs to be developed with the support of clinical professionals, community practitioners, and natural support systems; shared decision making is the best remedy possible. If you've never considered a Geriatric Care Manager before now, let me tell you a bit more about who they are and what they do.

A Geriatric Care Manager may provide the following duties (but not limited to):

Long-term Care Management

Long-term care management is assisting in the coordination of care for people living in a facility such as an assisted living or nursing facility.

A geriatric care manager might:

a. Provide quality of care visits and report significant concerns to the family

b. Assess the care plan developed by the facility and offer guidance on amendments, if warranted

c. Assess whether or not the facility is adhering to the care plan developed and approved

d. Act as the liaison between the facility, family, community resources and physicians

e. Advise the resident and family as to the resident's rights

Community Care Management

Community care management is assisting in the coordination of care for people living in the community in their own home or in the home of a family member or loved one.

A geriatric care manager might:

a. Conduct home visits

b. Perform a needs assessment for the person living with dementia

c. Assess the availability of community resources and make appropriate referrals

d. Develop a care plan for the senior and their family

e. Collaborate with the senior's physicians to coordinate medical care / planning

f. Make referrals to appropriate community based services and supports

g. Assistance in filing/appealing insurance forms/decisions

h. Consult with hospitals regarding discharge planning

i. Assist hospital or family in locating out-of-home placement, if warranted

j. Assess cognitive status

k. Assess eligibility for Medicaid or other forms of financial support

l. Assist family in obtaining Medicaid or other forms of financial support

m. Monitor quality of services provided

n. Act as a liaison between the senior, family, physicians, pharmacist, home care agencies, and other stakeholders

To locate a geriatric care manager near you, contact the Aging Life Care Association, https://aginglifecare.org.

*Two of the most important days of your life
is the day you find out what you love to do,
and the day you actually do it.*

Before the Diagnosis

Memory Loss

We typically identify memory loss as the one thing that defines a diagnosis of dementia. But the reality is that memory loss and lapses in judgement can be a normal part of aging; it's when these lapses pose a safety concern that we need to be concerned about.

Age-related memory loss is different from memory loss associated with various types of dementia, such as Alzheimer's disease, in that it doesn't significantly affect one's ability to carry out daily tasks. Occasionally forgetting where the keys are, walking into a room and forgetting why, or not being able to find the right words when having a conversation are all normal aging memory loss episodes and don't affect quality of life.

Unlike age-related memory loss, dementia is marked by a persistent, disabling decline in two or more intellectual abilities such as memory, language, judgment, and abstract thinking. Let me veer off for a moment here to talk about abstract thinking. Abstract thinking is the ability to think about and comprehend beyond what you see that is concrete. So, for example, if you tell someone with dementia to eat a banana; he/she might try to eat the banana without peeling it, because you said to "eat the banana;" you didn't say to peel the banana before you eat it. Someone who is an abstract thinker would know, without someone saying it, to peel the banana then eat it. Someone with advanced dementia might not be able to think beyond the concrete to understand the purpose of peeling the banana before eating it. Now, back to the point I was making about memory loss.

If you notice that your loved one is having increased frequency of these memory lapses, frequently repeating themselves, forgetting recent or routine information or are demonstrating increased agitation without a trigger, these could be signs of a more significant cognitive decline like dementia.

If you don't see your parents or older loved ones on a regular basis, you might notice a significant change from your last visit. If you see your parents more regularly, it's possible you may notice gradual changes over a period of time. One way to confirm your concerns is to talk to other family members and close friends to see if they have noticed similar changes. But keep in mind, if you have a concern, it is a valid concern and there is no harm in pursuing a consultation with your parent's primary care physician.

One thing I can't stress enough is that it's critical that you address any concerns with a medical provider as soon as you become aware of them. Early intervention for more serious cognitive decline is the best way to preserve quality of life
for your loved one.

It's important to acknowledge the emotions you may experience as you come to terms with what might be developing in your loved one: sadness, grief, fear, anger, hopelessness, and resentment. I encourage you to feel your feelings but don't allow them to prevent you from addressing the concerning behaviors you have noticed. There are many possible medical reasons for cognitive decline that are NOT dementia so don't think the worst from the very start. I encourage you to take a deep breath, acknowledge that you are taking positive action to promote quality of life for your loved one and take it one day at a time.

More Than Memory Loss

So, you've identified some concerning behaviors of your loved one that indicate something may be going on that is more serious than age-related memory loss. It's more than occasionally misplacing the phone, forgetting the name of a street or not being able to find the right word. You've noticed more frequent memory lapses, increased repetition and forgetfulness of new or routine information. It's now time to share those concerns with a medical professional.

Rather than raise the alarm with your loved one, casually ease into a discussion about it being time for an annual physical. You can offer to make the appointment. If your loved one doesn't take you up on that offer, you can wait a week or so and follow up to see if the appointment has been made. If it hasn't, go ahead and make the appointment. Whether you have made the appointment or not, it's a good idea to call the doctor's office prior to the appointment and let them know the reason for the visit. It is possible your parents won't disclose anything they have noticed about their memory loss or cognitive decline. If you live nearby, you can offer to drive. If you don't live nearby, arrange to be in town so you can go to the appointment, but try to make the visit under the guise of normal circumstances such as a vacation, holiday, or social visit.

It is helpful to not bring undue attention to your parents about their forgetful behaviors. It is likely they are aware on some level of their declines, and they are likely experiencing fear about the developments. Therefore, remain empathetic and try not to focus on it until a formal diagnosis has been made.

On the day of the appointment, help your loved one fill out the forms while in the waiting room. Ask your loved one to have you included on the HIPAA *(Health*

Information Portability & Accountability Act) form as someone with whom their medical information can be shared. This will facilitate your support and advocacy for your loved one and allow you to be a care partner.

Ideally, you would want to accompany your loved one into the exam room; however, if your parent declines to have you present during the doctor's visit, you can follow up with the doctor after the appointment. This is why calling ahead is so important, so the doctor is aware and can guide the conversation to where it needs to go.

At The Doctor's Appointment

First, I must tell you that there are many medical causes of dementia that are treatable. So, try to go into the appointment hoping for the best, but planning for the worst. One way to plan is by speaking with the doctor about treatable causes of dementia, such as a urinary tract infection, a vitamin B12 deficiency, thyroid imbalance, diabetes, medication interaction or side effect, depression or even a traumatic event like a death in the family. The doctor will first want to rule out any of these conditions so blood work will likely be ordered. But, let me warn you! The doctor might not order blood work. Therefore, you will need to advocate on your loved one's behalf by asking the doctor about the scenarios noted below.

Medications. Has your loved one started taking a new medication? Are there any side effects to the medications they are taking? Are there any interactions or contraindications between the medications (i.e., are the medications fighting against each other)? Are the 5 "Rights" being followed?

- The **Right** Person

- The **Right** Medication

- The **Right** Amount

- The **Right** Time

- The **Right** Route

I always encourage the use of one pharmacy; this way you can always go to the pharmacist to have a medication reconciliation performed to address potential issues with the medications prescribed. You simply ask the pharmacist to "check the medications for any adverse reactions." I tend to follow the path of least resistance here, as you will have a better chance of speaking with the pharmacist than you would have speaking with the person's doctor. You can also follow up with the nurse at the person's doctor's office.

Urinary Tract Infection. Does your loved one have a urinary tract infection (UTI)? A UTI is very common among the older population because they might not be as mobile as they used to be, they might not drink enough water or take in enough liquids, they might drink too much soda or caffeine *(our seniors tend to love soda and sweet* *tea)* or they might be incontinent. See my first book *A Dementia Caregiver's Guide to Care* for information on how to get your loved one to drink more water. You can thank me later!

You will want to request a urinalysis from a medical professional and have positive results prior to taking any antibiotics. In the event you would like to assess the likelihood of a UTI prior to seeing a medical professional, you can purchase a urinary screening kit from your local pharmacy. The kit is for "screening" purposes only and not a diagnostic tool. The test will only provide information that may suggest if the person might have a UTI. If the test is positive that means you should follow up with their physician as soon as possible.

Dehydration. Is your loved one dehydrated? As we get older, our body's thirst signal tends to diminish over time. That's why older adults and seniors tend to not drink a lot of water. As a result, the chances of dehydration occurring is very high. Dehydration can wreak havoc on a senior's psyche if not treated. It can cause severe delirium, confusion, behavioral changes, aggression, agitation, and depressive symptoms. If you suspect dehydration, please seek medical attention immediately.

Nutritional Imbalance. Is your loved one deprived of essential nutrients, such as vitamin B, vitamin D, or vitamin E? These vitamins are essential in maintaining brain health. Therefore, you should have a medical professional complete laboratory tests to make the determination as to whether the person is lacking any essential vitamins. The lack of vitamin B12 is one area I tend to see a lot in the older population. If the person has a vitamin B12 deficiency, the doctor might prescribe B12 tablets or even a B12 shot; vitamin supplements may also be prescribed. Although the supplements can be purchased over the counter, I highly recommend the doctor still prescribe the over the counter (OTC) medications to better manage the side effects, if any.

Lack of Sleep. How often is your loved one sleeping? Is your loved one sleeping at night or are they sleeping more during the day? It is important that your loved one gets the proper amount of sleep: 6 – 9 hours are recommended for adults. But the fact of the matter is that those living with dementia may not get that many hours at night because they might sleep continually throughout the day. I know you might be saying that as long as they are sleeping, what's the problem? Day sleeping becomes a concern when the caregiver has to be up at night with the person after working all day; this scenario does not bode well for either party because of the agitation, anxiety, stress, and frustration that will be exhibited on both sides. When this occurs, quality of care and the quality of life for the caregiver and their loved one is severely impacted. This is where developing a routine would come in handy. Develop a sleep schedule and ensure meaningful activities are made available for your loved one throughout the day so that he/she will be tired at night and more apt to go to sleep and to stay asleep.

Depression. Has there been a major life event, such as a death in the family? Is your loved one extremely sad about the death? If so, the person might be depressed. It might not be dementia at all. It is important to note that depression can be treated, even in older adults; but you have to report any life changes to the doctor, including irregular sleeping patterns or if they are not sleeping at all. These conditions can be treated, and if treated properly, you may see the dementia symptoms go away. But, if the symptoms don't resolve, there might be an even bigger problem to address.

Should the doctor rule out any of the conditions noted above as the reason for the memory loss, he or she may then assess your loved one using a conversation tool called the Informant Questionnaire on Cognitive Decline. This tool will help the doctor establish baseline information, along with the patient's medical history. This is one reason why seeing the primary care physician is important; he/she knows your loved one and their history. The next step should be a referral to a neurologist for a cognitive test and brain scans that can determine if the cause is a particular type of dementia. So, be sure to ask for information and resources to help you gain a better understanding of the disease your loved one might have and how it will progress.

The Diagnosis

What to Expect

If your loved one does indeed have dementia, you may experience some intense emotions. While the diagnosis may be scary and devastating, it's important to note that you have helped your loved one get an early jump on a progressive disease which will help preserve their quality of life to the greatest extent possible. Keeping a positive attitude and leading with compassion will allow you to continue in your role as supporter, advocate and care partner.

Many are fearful of what's to come after there is a "diagnosis" of dementia. But there is so much to unpack here. First, I put DIAGNOSIS in parentheses because dementia is not a diagnosis – it is a symptom of a disease or condition. Doctors will often use the term dementia as the diagnosis which does cause some confusion for those who know the difference between a diagnosis and a symptom. So, let me back up a little to my first book when I talked about the different types or causes of dementia. There are more than 100 causes of dementia – the most common cause is Alzheimer's disease. The second most common cause of dementia is vascular disease typically caused by stroke activity. Having several mini strokes can cause vascular dementia. Then there's Dementia with Lewy Bodies, Frontotemporal Dementia, HIV or AIDS associated dementia, and the list goes on and on.

Dementia is the symptom or symptoms of having a condition that impairs one's cognitive abilities. For example, if you go to the doctor for a headache, when your examination is complete, the doctor is going to write what's causing the headache, such as an upper respiratory infection and you may receive medication to treat the underlying cause of the headache (i.e., the infection) and you may even receive medication to treat the symptoms (i.e., the headache).

Well, treating dementia is the same way; the only difference is, for now, there is no treatment, cure or preventative measures for the underlying condition (i.e. Alzheimer's). However, there are treatment options for many of the symptoms of dementia which may include confusion, disorientation, forgetfulness, irritability, agitation, aggression and lack of judgement.

After The Diagnosis

Common Questions

Once a family receives a diagnosis of a progressive type of dementia like Alzheimer's disease, a barrage of questions consumes their thinking.

- *What type of care will my loved one need?*

- *When do I move them in with me?*

- *When do I move them into a facility?*

- *Will they remember me?*

- *Who will take care of them when I'm working?*

- *Will I need to stop working?*

- *Will I need to leave my family to move to where they live?*

- *Why am I so angry? I love my parents.*

- *Why am I so frustrated and feeling burdened? I enjoy taking care of my parents.*

To have these types of questions enter your mind after the diagnosis is perfectly normal and we will get to them all. But, first, let's address the emotional piece of caring for someone with a life limiting, brain robbing illness such as dementia. Caring for a family member can be very rewarding, but the 1 in 5 Americans who do so on a daily basis can promise you that it's not always easy. There are a lot of emotions involved and sometimes they can get in the way of life. These emotions include anger, resentment, guilt, sadness, grief, worry and loneliness.

Anger

Anger often comes from a sense of obligation or a sense of being taken for granted. Caregivers can feel as though they're stuck with the biggest workload because they're the oldest sibling, they're closest to the one receiving care or no one else is around to help. On the outside looking in, it's hard for someone else to understand the time and effort you're putting in, and that can trigger anger in a caregiver.

Resentment

Feeling resentment is like feeling anger, but not quite the same. Clinicians label this feeling as "the re-experiencing of past wrongdoings, real or perceived," a feeling that you're stuck in servitude of the person causing your discomfort. This means resentment is often aimed at the person you're caring for, as their aging process or illness creates more responsibilities for you and makes you take on an additional role on top of your everyday life.

Guilt

Guilt is a particularly draining emotion, and it typically comes after noticing feelings of anger and resentment.

Once you reflect on your emotions and begin to feel bad that you've developed hostile feelings towards a loved one, guilt is the next logical response. It can also be a primary driver of caregiver stress and burnout, as many family caregivers feel guilty for needing a break or not being able to do more for a loved one.

Sadness

On the surface, sadness is much easier to notice as a family caregiver. Watching a loved one age or decline from illness can take a profound toll and make you feel an imminent sense of loss and eventual depression. Caregivers can also feel sadness once they start to miss their old life, before the stress and responsibilities caused by taking care of someone else.

Grief

Grief is a much deeper sense of sadness that a caregiver may not be able to fully understand right away. In addition to feeling sadness about impending loss, a caregiver may feel grief about already losing who they felt their loved one was before an illness. In extreme cases, a caregiver may also feel grief as if they've lost a part of themselves. Watching a loved one decline is mentally and emotionally draining; it's a process that can forever alter who you are going forward. Feeling grief from this is a perfectly normal response.

Worry

All of the emotions mentioned above contribute to a sense of worry and anxiety, for not only your loved one but also yourself and the rest of your family. Being a family caregiver can make you concerned about some obvious things, such as your loved one's well-being and future. But it can also make you question how your family dynamic will be changed, if you might have a similar future to the person you're caring for, how the financials of the situation will play out and overall anxiety about anything else that can go wrong.

Loneliness

When a caregiver begins to notice this range of emotions, they often isolate themselves and experience a feeling of loneliness. Not only do caregivers have less time to get out and socialize or do the things they enjoy, but it can also be difficult to share your struggle with others. Many times, caregivers fear being judged for struggling to help a loved one, or they simply don't want others to know that their loved one is in a state of decline. By hiding these struggles, it amplifies the sense of isolation from friends and other family members.

It's possible that caregivers may be unaware of the exact emotion they are feeling. That's why taking the time for some self-reflection or conversation with a trusted friend or family member can help you understand your emotions and why you are experiencing them. I always like to say you can't fix what you don't face.

Once you can name the emotion, give yourself permission to feel it. It's ok to have these feelings. They are real and valid. But the danger here is that if these emotions remain unchecked, it may have a negative effect on the person receiving care. Just remember that managing these emotions paves the way for person-centered care to be front and center – the desired approach to optimizing quality of life and positive outcomes for those we care for.

Planning for Care

The doctors have confirmed it, your mom or dad has a progressive type of dementia. But the reality is that dementia is not just an individual diagnosis, it is a family diagnosis. The road forward is one you and your loved one will take together. It may be hard for you not to take charge, but I want to assure you that walking side by side as care partners will result in far better outcomes for everyone.

So, what's the dynamic at play here? As the adult child of a parent with newly diagnosed dementia, you likely have been working for many years, have a lot of experience and may even be at the top of your career. You may feel the need to lead the charge with your parents. You may feel like it's not only your natural inclination ingrained from your job experience, but your familial duty to take care of your parents as they took care of you. Both responses are natural but unfortunately neither approach is fully effective because it removes the locus of control from your parent. In short, this approach compromises your parents' fiercely guarded independence, which they now know is in jeopardy.

Assuming an authoritative role in the care of your parent with dementia is threatening. And when people are threatened, they often become resistant and even uncooperative in an effort to retain independence – an unintended consequence of your good intentions to help. Put yourself in your parents' shoes and I'm sure you can understand and empathize with the flurry of emotions that accompany a diagnosis of dementia: fear, sadness, shame, anger, hopelessness. Instead adopt a collaborative approach. This will improve cooperation and adoption of changes put in place to help your parents live their best life. And at the end of the day, that is the outcome everyone wants. Your aging loved one has been diagnosed with a condition that leads to dementia. Now is a good time to begin advanced care planning with your loved one.

An early diagnosis of dementia gives you and your loved one time to make plans before their decision-making abilities are affected. Consider the following:

Enlist an Attorney

One of the first things to do when starting advanced care planning is to secure an elder care attorney. This professional will be well-versed in drawing up important documents such as a Durable Power of Attorney and a Health Care Power of Attorney. These documents outline who is responsible for making financial and health related decisions in the event your loved one is unable to. These documents are particularly important when dealing with a progressive disease that results in cognitive decline. It's important to note that if these documents aren't in place, the Adult Health Care Consent Act dictates who the decision maker will be typically starting with spouse, then children from oldest to youngest.

Become a Co-Signer on Financial Documents

With your loved one's consent, a responsible party should become a co-signer on any back accounts, pension plans or other financial documents. This allows you to become familiar with your loved one's assets, understand what needs to be managed and how money is dispersed while your loved one is still able to be involved.

Stay on Top of Bills

As your loved one's cognitive abilities decline, they also may experience diminished executive functioning which is the ability to get things done. They may forget to pay the electricity bill or order winter fuel and find themselves sitting in the dark or freezing cold. You can work with your loved one to gain online access to accounts and automate payments, if desired. Adding your email to their account is useful in case passwords are forgotten.

Make a List of Medical Providers

From the primary care physician to the pharmacy to any specialists your loved one sees, it's a good idea to know all the players on the care team. Your loved one will be living with dementia, but other health issues are likely to arise. It's also important to have your loved one add you to the HIPAA form so that you have access to their medical information.

Partnering with your loved one on advanced care planning is a great way to preserve their independence and dignity and ensures that when the time comes, you will be able to take care of them to your best ability.

Types of Care

As noted above, one of the questions that you might have is, "What type of care will my loved one need?" The short answer is that the level of care depends on the person's age and the disease stage. There are five prominent stages of the disease process. Below are the symptoms that may be displayed during the various stages of the disease.

Early stages of dementia might reveal the following symptoms:

- Recent Memory loss

- Word-find difficulties

- Poor judgment

- Poor decision making

- Time/place disorientation

- Depression

- Apathy

- Difficulty performing familiar / simple tasks

- Needing reminders about important dates, people, and places and how to perform familiar tasks, such as making a cup of coffee

- Decreased concentration

- Difficulty following conversations

- Communication may be disjointed or facts are distorted

- Forgetting parts and pieces of experiences (i.e. retiring from work)

- Misplacing things and blaming you for stealing them

Middle stages of dementia might reveal the following symptoms:

- Risk to self/unsafe to be left alone

- Increased memory loss

- Mood disturbances

- Increased word-find difficulties

- Problems tracking conversations

- Calculation difficulty

- Reading may stop

- Visual-spatial perception problems *(unable to visually process letters, words)*

- Repetitive behaviors

- Inability to recognize familiar faces

- Hyperorality *(inserting inappropriate items in mouth)*

Later stages of dementia might reveal the following symptoms:

- Behavioral outbursts

- Depression

- Paranoia/hallucination

- Getting lost in familiar place, such as their home or neighborhood

- Wandering away

- Considerable weight loss

- Increased risk for falls

- Incontinence

- Needs hands on assistance with their activities of daily living (i.e. bathing, dressing, toileting, grooming, oral hygiene)

- Requires simplified instructions to complete basic tasks due to the lack of abstract thinking abilities

- Loss of inhibition; therefore, they may say what comes to mind (i.e. what comes up, comes out)

End of Life stages of dementia might reveal the following symptoms:

- Unable to perform activities of daily living independently

- Immobility

- Inability to perform purposeful movement

- Swallowing difficulties

- Fragile skin

- Limited communication

- Non-verbal

Keeping the above stages above in mind, you want to be sure you are giving the right type of care at the right time. Give the care they need, not the care you think they need or that you want to give them to reduce your burden.

In-home Care Options

Now that the diagnosis has been confirmed by a team of medical professionals, your mind begins to wonder about how long your loved one should remain in their home alone. The good thing is that the disease does not progress to its worst overnight. Therefore, you have time to plan. Of course, our older family members won't come right out and tell us they need help, as they fear they may lose their independence. That's why I recommend engaging them in casual conversation that takes into consideration their feelings.

Below are four main areas to assess to determine if additional help is warranted:

Activities of Daily Living

If they are having trouble completing simple tasks, such as making a bed or making a pot of coffee, there may be some physical decline. You can take note of their appearance: Are their clothes clean? Do they match? Are they bathing? If it appears that they have lost some weight, ask them about what they have been eating lately. This can tell you if they are having trouble food shopping or cooking. I would also say that a noticeable loss of weight is a definite cause for concern as it could indicate an underlying health condition.

The Home Environment

Check to see if the home is more cluttered than usual. This could be a sign they are having trouble keeping up with housekeeping. You can also check the refrigerator to get a sense of how well they are eating. Additionally, take a look at the expiration dates on the medicine bottles and appropriately discard any expired medications – prescription as well as over the counter ones. You'd want to throw away any expired food items, as well.

Mobility

Take note of how they move about the house. Are they grabbing onto furniture to steady themselves? Do you notice any bruising which may indicate a recent fall? Go on a walk with them to see if they tire easily or seem unbalanced. In addition, understanding their driving habits may be helpful. Look at their car for any dents, dings, or scratches, as this could be an indication that they are having concerns with driving.

Social Engagement

Ask about friends they are in touch with either in person or on the phone, as well as any regular activities or recent outings. Are there activities they have stopped doing? Are there things they wish they could do but don't have a companion or a ride?

Before you consider moving your loved one from his/her home, you should know that in the early stages of the disease process, your loved one may only need a few reminders to keep them as independent as they possibly can. So, try writing things down, like names, numbers, appointments in big letters w/ colors contrasting (black background with white letters tends to pop) so that your loved one can easily read and connect with the information. Adding pictures may also help as the disease progresses; for example, putting a picture of a toilet on the bathroom door.

As the disease progresses, there will be moments and areas of concern. If you ever become concerned about health and/or safety, such as leaving the stove on or wandering away from home and getting lost or messing up on taking medications, it might be time to consider additional support. Many times, seniors don't want to leave their home, so try bringing in someone to assist them in their own home.

When considering in-home care options, there are few things you want to look out for and/or ask:

- How to get started?

- Is there a non-refundable deposit?

- What are the back-up care options in the event the in-home caregiver calls out?

- How do you accept payments?

- Is there a minimum number of days?

- Is there a minimum number of hours per day?

- How often are the in-home caregivers trained?

- Are they trained in dementia competent practices?

- What dementia curriculum are they trained in?

- How often are they trained/retrained?

- Is there an opportunity for cross training family caregivers to be able to manage the care when the in-home caregiver is not there?

- Is there an emergency plan in place if the in-home caregiver is needed outside of regular contracted hours?

- Will we have the same in-home caregiver every day?

You might also find that the senior might not be receptive to receiving "help." So, you might try using a different term. You might say that someone is coming to clean for them or that you've arranged for a personal assistant, and that they are in charge of the person and would need to tell them what to do. In the meantime, you would have already told the in-home caregiver what the deal was so that she/he can go along with the plan. This puts control back into the hands of the senior who now might be more receptive to receiving care. This is what we had to do with my grandma who had dementia. She actually fired the in-home caregiver that we hired so we had to bring in my sister, her granddaughter that she raised, to provide support in her home.

Now that wasn't all that easy either. My grandma didn't want my sister to miss work to help her. What my grandma didn't realize was that my sister's "work" was as an in-home caregiver so this was what she did for a living; but my grandma still wouldn't go for it. So, we told her that my sister wasn't working at the moment, so she had time to give back to her what my grandma had given to her. She went for that, and it made her feel so good.

You will also need to evaluate and assess the in-home caregiver that will help your loved one. Consider the following characteristics when interviewing potential in-home caregivers:

- **Sincerity** – Caregivers genuinely care about the people they care for and have a desire to make their lives as comfortable and enjoyable as possible. This compassion is one of the defining characteristics of a caregiver.

- **Competency** – People receiving care may be scared or insecure about their need for care so it's helpful to reassure them by exhibiting confidence and competence. If a person believes in your abilities, they will feel more secure, safe and engaged.

- **Committed** – Good caregivers advocate for their clients. They ask questions and expect answers. They also learn about their condition so they can provide the most appropriate care.

- **Uplifting** – Caregivers understand that there will be good days and bad days. They try to focus on the positive and find the silver lining in every situation. This positive outlook is contagious and can often help the people they're caring for feel better about themselves.

- **Collaborative** – A good caregiver recognizes that they are part of an extended care team that may include doctors, family and friends. Being understanding and flexible goes a long way toward being a successful team player focused on what's best for the person receiving care.

- **Patience** – This is the most important because it is key to providing a safe and comfortable atmosphere. People who need care often take longer to complete simple tasks, and they may ask the same questions over and over. Quality caregivers need patience to deal with anything from a loved one's memory lapses to angry outbursts. They must practice staying calm and avoid frustration.

Caregivers likely will not be exhibiting all of these characteristics at once. Instead, they draw on the appropriate quality based on the situation. Having a well-stocked caregiving toolbox is invaluable for caregivers.

Live-In Care Options

If you're wondering if it's time to make alternative living arrangements for your loved one, including bringing in someone to live with them in their home, having them live with a relative, or having them live with you, consider the following:

- Do they need 24-hour supervision?

- Do they wander?

- Do they leave the stove on?

- Do they forget to take their medications?

- Do they forget to eat?

If you answered yes to most of the questions above, it might be time to begin planning for an alternative living arrangement for your loved one.

Now, before you contemplate having your loved one with dementia live with you and your family, here are a few things you should consider:

- Do you have the space for them to have their own area?

- Are you willing to be flexible and step into their reality?

- Do you have the patience to provide care?

- Do you have the ability to not control them and tell them what to do?

- Are you willing to partner in their care and support their decisions, within reason?

- If you're working, do you plan to stop working?

Do you have family members and friends who can help you with care? Would you trust someone you don't know to come into your home to care for your loved one while you work or need a break?

If your response is "*no*" to most of these questions, then it might be time to consider out-of-home/facility care. Of the questions listed, the most telling questions are the ones about paying for in-home care, working, and having family members/friends to help you, as the types of long-term services and supports are very few and far in between.

Let's define what long-term care and long-term support services (LTSS) are. LTSS and long-term care are typically non-medical supportive services one may need on a longer-term basis, such as assistance with activities of daily living (i.e. bathing, dressing, eating, etc.), assisted living care, nursing home care, and/or adult day health/care.

Cost of Long-Term Care

The conundrum is that the cost of long-term care can have an astronomical price tag. There once was a sense of comfort knowing that when one reaches the age of 65,

Medicare will provide for most, if not all long-term care needs. The reality is that Medicare does not cover long-term care services and support (LTSS). The amount of care that a senior may need as they age will depend on the type and amount of financial resources they have.

Because of the limited financial resources that are available to pay for the long-term care services for seniors, family members bear the brunt of the responsibility for providing that care, which is not an easy feat as long-term care that involves out-of-home placement, such as assisted living or skilled nursing facilities, can cost anywhere from $4,000 to $10,000 per month. Long term care services that are provided within the home, such as having a professional caregiver come into the home to assist with activity of daily living, supervision and companionship, can cost anywhere from $15 - $28 per hour, which can quickly add up if a loved one needs care every day for most of the day. Based on my experience, family members tend to look at their loved one's finances first, and when they realize their loved one would go bankrupt if they paid for their own care, they tend to look at their own finances to figure out how to supplement the cost of care. And that's where we look at alternative options.

There are a few options that I recommend when looking at alternatives to paying for long-term services and supports. Your loved one can sell their home and use the cash to pay for their care. You can enlist the help of an elder attorney to do Medicaid planning for your loved one, even if they have already been diagnosed. Or you can look into your loved one getting a whole life insurance policy.

While more than 50% of individuals over the age of 65 have some type of life insurance, it's important to note that not all life insurance policies are created equal. There is a difference between term life insurance and whole life insurance. Term life insurance provides coverage for a specified period (the term of the policy) and includes a death benefit; whereas whole life insurance is lifelong coverage that includes a death benefit and typically has a cash value account that builds interest.

I highly recommend contacting a licensed whole life insurance advisor to weigh your loved one's options. This might also help you plan for your own care as you get older. When you meet with the advisor about your loved one, be open to alternatives and ask lots of questions to ensure all your concerns are addressed to your satisfaction. And be sure to inquire about the benefits and risks and how the death benefit will be affected if there are any withdrawals or loans on the cash value savings account. Taking this information into consideration will better prepare you to make an informed decision about planning for long-term care for your loved one.

Long-Term Care Options

Now that you know a little bit more about long-term services and supports, what is covered and what is considered out of pocket costs, let's look at what to expect from various long-term care options.

Nursing Home / Skilled Nursing Facility (SNF)

- These facilities provide 24-hour nursing and rehabilitation for people who have chronic medical conditions or impaired mental capacity and who have significant deficiencies in performing their activities of daily living.

Assisted Living Community (ALC)

- An ALC provides care for individuals who need some help with activities of daily living (ADLs) yet wish to remain as independent as possible.

- This is a middle ground between independent living and nursing homes.

- Most facilities offer 24-hour supervision, most often by non-licensed staff, and an array of support services that may include medication management and memory care services.

Continuing Care Retirement Community (CCRC) or Life Care Facility

- CCRCs offer independent and assisted living, as well as medical and nursing services up to and including SNF care.

- Residents progress to the level of care they need.

- Some CCRCs also offer special-care units.

Senior housing

- Under the Fair Housing Act, "housing for older persons" is housing that is specifically designed for occupation by elderly people under a federal, state, or local government program.

- This type of housing is occupied solely by people who are 62 or older.

- Senior housing houses at least one person who is 55 or older in at least 80% of the occupied units.

- Benefits to senior housing may include proximity to shopping or medical facilities, security features, safety-equipped units, community activities and transportation.

Adult Day Care

- Adult day-care centers can offer supervision, social and recreational activities, lunch, and possibly health-related oversight during the day for adults who may need care outside of the home or residential care facility.

*Sidebar: **Aging Alone***

There are many seniors with no family at all – no spouse/partner, no children, no siblings, no one to help them as their needs progress. With that mind, although we're talking about caring for a loved one with dementia, aging without family is a real concern that comes with a few challenges that I want to prepare you for, as well. Here are a few things you might want to consider for yourself and for those you know with no family support as it relates to residential options.

- ***Long-term care insurance*** *may cover costs for home care aides or help afford assisted living.*

- ***Shared housing*** *matches people who have unused space with people who need housing; typically, at least one party is age 60 or older. The people with extra living space typically want company, help around the house or extra income or sometimes all three.*

- ***Co-housing*** *is a living arrangement created by its residents so they can live together in small homes, using a common house for meals, meetings, and activities to foster social connection and support.*

- *The **village movement**, typically a non-profit grassroots membership organization that coordinates a variety of services like transportation, home repair and maintenance, and social engagement opportunities, to name a few. The basic premise behind the village* *movement is the opportunity for seniors to remain in their own home as opposed to living in an assisted living community or senior housing.*

Now, back to what I was saying about moving into a long-term care community. When considering nursing home or assisted living options, you want to be prepared to inquire about the following:

- Is there a special area for people living with dementia?

- Do they have to wear monitors on their ankles? *(I am completely against this. If this is happening run far and wide away from this facility.)*

- How long have staff been employed?

- How often are staff trained in dementia competent practices?

- Ask to see the training curriculum. It should not be a FAQ sheet that employees sign. Staff need to be sitting in a training, either face to face or virtually, on a routine basis.

- How often are staff trained and retrained in dementia competent care?

- What activities will residents participate in?

- Do residents have to eat in the dining room with everyone else every day for every meal? Can they eat in their room?

- What is your process if residents refuse to take a bath, eat or take their medications?

- What is your process if residents refuse to participate in an activity?

Behavioral Considerations

As you consider any of the changes in living arrangements mentioned above, you want to be mindful of the behaviors associated with progressive types of dementia that may pose challenges at any stage of the disease process. A few of the most common behaviors that are considered challenging when it comes to caring for someone with dementia are as follows:

- Agitation

- Physical and verbal aggression

- Repetition (doing and saying things over and over again)

- Rummaging (moving things from one area to the next and building clutter)

- Wandering

These behaviors may be caused by several things other than dementia. The list below will provide guidance on things that might cause someone with dementia to display challenging behaviors:

Physical Causes of Concerning Behavior

- Pain/Discomfort

    - The person might be in pain or experiencing discomfort due to a medical condition or surgeries (sometimes even previous surgeries performed years ago.)

- Medications

    - As mentioned earlier, the person's medications might be causing side effects, such as irritability, aggression, agitation, and anxiety. The medications he/she is taking might also be "fighting" against each other, meaning one medication might be causing the other one not to work properly.

- Thirst / Hunger

    - They may be thirsty or hungry and do not know how to verbally express what they desire. Therefore, they use what they still have full access to and that is aggressive behavior, but it's only to get your attention since we tend to respond quickly to something that's negative, bothersome, or disturbing. But please know that the person is not intentionally being mean or hateful to you; it's just the only thing they know how to do to get your attention to get their needs met.

- Acute illness

- Also, mentioned earlier, the person could have a urinary tract infection (UTI) which causes significant behavior challenges such as delirium, confusion, memory loss, and sometimes aggression and wandering.

- Lack of sleep

  - They could be tired because they are not sleeping well at night. Not having a good night's sleep will cause anyone to be irritable or short tempered and agitated.

Cognitive Causes of Concerning Behavior

- They may not be able to understand what you or others are trying to communicate; therefore, they are misunderstood and overlooked.

- They may be frustrated because they cannot remember things they want to remember or things you think they should remember.

- They may be dealing with hearing or vision loss; and that's why they are not doing what you ask them to do. They can't pick up something they don't see or didn't hear you say. Be sure to have their hearing and vision checked out on an annual basis with their physical exam.

Emotional Causes of Concerning Behavior

- Fear tends to cause people with dementia to have behavioral responses that are not favorable. They are afraid of what's happening to them and what's happening around them. Just know that they have been experiencing dementia symptoms way before anyone else noticed, to the sum of about 15 – 20 years before diagnosis. So, much of the behaviors you see is the person fighting for control and independence over their own life.

Environmental Causes of Concerning Behavior

- There is too much noise (over stimulation) or not enough noise (under stimulation). Think about the type of work your loved one did prior to dementia. If they were in a choir or band, they would probably love to have music in their space. If they were a librarian, they probably would appreciate the peace and quiet. It's very important to know who they were before the disease developed so that you can plan and prepare their environment.

- The home that they live in is no longer familiar to them. Since people with dementia tend to remember a long time ago and experience trouble remembering recent information, the home that they lived in for the past 20 years is no longer their home and they want to go home, and they might begin to wander.

I know you've heard that line before, "I want to go home." And you sometimes say, "You are home." Well, their current home is not the home they are talking about; they are talking about their childhood home with their parents and siblings. Of course, they can no longer go back there, but you can talk with them about the good old days and reminisce. That should take their mind off going back home, at least for a moment.

Caregiver Communication Causes of Concerning Behavior

- The caregiver is rushing the person to do something, such as getting dressed or eating.

- The caregiver is too aggressive in his/her tone when talking to the person, such as saying mean words or sounding mean in his/her tone of voice.

- The caregiver is not talking slow enough for the person to understand what the caregiver is trying to say.

- There are too many people telling the person what to do and each of them is using different words, phrases, tones of voice, and body language and this causes confusion for the person.

Am I talking about you without calling your name? Do you fit the description of any of these points? If so, you've made the first step and that is identifying that you are contributing to the concerning behavior the person is displaying. Now, here are some practical tips for you to begin to incorporate into your day-to-day care routine.

Practical Solutions to Reducing Concerning Behaviors

- Allow the person to do things that are familiar to him/her, such as wiping down the table after dinner or sweeping the floor or taking out the trash. This would be so meaningful.

- Use appropriate communication skills by giving them short instructions and one at a time, such as "stand up," "walk over here," "sit down here," "pick up your spoon," "put it in the rice," "pick up the spoon," "open your mouth," "put the spoon in your mouth."

- Congratulate them on completing a task, as opposed to criticizing them, even if it is not to the caregiver's liking. For example, if they put their shirt on inside out, don't say that it's on backwards, say that they did a good job putting on their shirt.

- Don't surprise them when talking to them about doing something. Caregivers should approach them from the front, but at an angle. Then, they should establish a connection with the person with a simple greeting or a conversation about the weather. After the connection is established, the caregiver can then discuss with them the next step.

- Give them appropriate choices and try not to control their decisions. Making decisions helps to promote independence. The choices that you provide them need to be appropriate, though. For example, if it's 100 degrees outside, the choice of clothing should be two outfits that are worn in the summertime (i.e. short sleeves) as opposed to the winter (i.e. long sleeves). So, no matter what they choose, it will be appropriate.

- Keep the environment simple and calm. Don't overwhelm them with lots of colors and patterns on the floor and walls (i.e., decorative pictures and patterned rugs).

- Establish a predictable routine with them and stick to the routine so they know what to do next and won't have to ask you repeatedly, because I know how much you love that!

- Minimize change in the people who come in to provide care and support. Remember, routine is key and that includes people, too.

Resources

Alzheimer's disease has been identified as a public health emergency and not a normal part of aging. Detecting the disease in the early stages is sometimes difficult because of the similarities to normal aging. Therefore, learning the signs and symptoms of the disease process is paramount to the health of the person living with dementia and their caregivers. Connecting people to resources has always been my superpower. As a social worker, I am outcomes oriented and solutions focused. So, let me connect you to some resources that I have found especially helpful in my personal journey through dementia with my grandma and in my professional career as a dementia specialist caring for and guiding families through this maze of care.

#1 Geriatric Care Practice (Medical)

- Find a geriatric care practice, sometimes called a senior primary care practice. This type of medical group will not only have geriatricians – doctors specializing in the care of older adults – it will also have licensed social workers, gerontologists, community health liaisons and health care advocates all working together to connect its patients to the services they need.

#2 Area Agency on Aging (Social)

- You should also seek out your local <u>Area Agency on Aging</u>. This agency is designated by the state to address the needs and concerns of all senior citizens at regional and local levels.

#3 Certified Elder Care Attorney (Legal)

- Another great resource is an elder care attorney who handles a wide range of legal matters concerning older adults. These include the creation of living wills, advanced care directives and long-term care planning.

Above, I've covered all the essential aspects of care from medical care to social care to legal care. Next, I'm connecting you to all things in between:

1. **Alzheimer's Association**

   - Education

   - Respite

   - Support Groups

     https://www.alz.org/

2. **National Institute on Aging: Alzheimer's Caregiving Tips**

   - Education

     https://www.nia.nih.gov/health/alzheimers-caregiving

3. **Elder Care Locator**

- Connecting seniors and caregivers to local support by ZIP code

  https://eldercare.acl.gov/

4. **Nursing Home Compare**

- Locate Medicare-certified nursing homes in your area based on ZIP code

- Access Medicare-certified nursing home quality of care reports and staffing break down

  https://www.medicare.gov/what-medicare-covers/what-part-a-covers/compare-nursing-home-quality

5. ***Joy For All* Companion Pets**

- Robotic companion pets

- Nostalgic board games for each generation

  https://joyforall.com/

6. **The Alzheimer's Store**

- Dementia vetted products for all stages

- Wandering prevention products

- Dementia friendly games & activities

- Nostalgic products

  https://www.alzstore.com/

Congratulations! You've made it this far and guess what? You're now better prepared today than you were yesterday and the day before and the day before. So, what's next? What's next is what's happening now. Now, you're putting supports and strategies in place to assist you in taking care of your loved one and YOU, for the duration of this caregiving journey.

But it doesn't stop there. It is now incumbent upon you to share what you've learned with someone else who is going through or about to go through what you're experiencing. You are well positioned to do just that and to afford your loved one the quality of living they so rightly deserve, minding what matters most.

Although there's not a cure, there is care. YOUR CARE!